YOUR KNOWLEDGE HAS VALUE

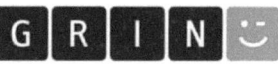

Bibliographic information published by the German National Library:

The German National Library lists this publication in the National Bibliography;
detailed bibliographic data are available on the Internet at http://dnb.dnb.de .

Imprint:

Copyright © 2015 GRIN Verlag, Open Publishing GmbH
Print and binding: Books on Demand GmbH, Norderstedt Germany
ISBN: 978-3-668-15114-7

Hariesh Rajasekar

A Brief Report on Data Breaches in U.S. Healthcare. What, Why, and How?

GRIN Publishing

GRIN - Your knowledge has value

Since its foundation in 1998, GRIN has specialized in publishing academic texts by students, college teachers and other academics as e-book and printed book. The website www.grin.com is an ideal platform for presenting term papers, final papers, scientific essays, dissertations and specialist books.

Visit us on the internet:

http://www.grin.com/

http://www.facebook.com/grincom

http://www.twitter.com/grin_com

A Brief Report on Data Breaches in U.S. Healthcare – What, Why, and How?

Hariesh Rajasekar*
* MS Health Informatics,
Bouvé College of Health Sciences,
Northeastern University,
Boston, Massachusetts, USA.

Hariesh Rajasekar

Abstract:

Data breaches in U.S. healthcare have become ubiquitous with modern hackers honing in on healthcare data due to its lucrative economic value. Cyber crooks regard medical identity theft as **'The triple crown of stolen data'** as it's worth more than a Social Security Number or credit card number in the internet black market. The black market rate for each partial EHR is $50 as compared to $1 for a stolen Social Security Number or credit card number. With 44% of data breaches that healthcare organizations contribute to, this report analyzes for the evolving security measures and trends in the healthcare industry to protect data from cyber crooks. An infographic study was carried out to explore the ways by which data is lost, states accounting the most and least number of medical data breaches, and the location of breached information. Outcome of this infographics study is expected to pave the way for possibility of future research and scholarly debate. Potential of cloud computing in healthcare has been taken into account and was analyzed for its benefits of adoption and use, obstacles, and its forecast in the near future. At the outset, this report is a snapshot of U.S. healthcare's defensive preparation and strategy against the level of cyber-attacks that will be coming at them, statistical analysis on types of breach impacting healthcare organizations the most, state-wise percentage analysis of medical data breach, and cloud computing as a defensive solution to protect the data from cyber-attacks, and insider threat - disgruntled employees and patient-record snoopers.

Keywords: Medical ID theft, economic value, cyber threats, breach types, defensive strategies, cloud computing.

Hariesh Rajasekar

Table of Contents

Introduction:

Information security (InfoSec) is critical to every organization today – especially healthcare, with the reports of breaches against healthcare organizations, large and small, continuing to rise.[1] That said, International Data Corporation (IDC) predicts 1 out of 3 individuals will have their healthcare records compromised by cyber-attacks in 2016.[2] Modern hackers of the online world regard medical information as a **'treasure trove'** given its lucrative economic value.[3] Large amounts of credential information including, name, birth date, policy number, diagnostic code(s), billing information, and Social Security Numbers contained in the Electronic Health Record make it worth the trouble for the hackers.[4]

The potential of granular data is certainly propelling hackers of all stripes to perforate the defenses of hospitals and other health organizations holding such data. The healthcare industry in particular is an enticing target to data breach as the market for stolen medical records continue to grow.[5] These records are auctioned and sold in remote corners of the internet black market. Medical and personnel records are increasingly valuable to cybercriminals than credit card data.[6] According to FBI, the black market rate for each partial EHR is $50 as compared to $1 for a stolen Social Security Number or credit card number.[7] Some of the notable data breaches in healthcare between 2009 and 2015 is shown in **Figure 1.**

[1] Hourihan, C., Cline, B. (2012, December). *A look back: U.S. healthcare data breach trends*. Retrieved from https://hitrustalliance.net/content/uploads/2014/05/HITRUST-Report-U.S.-Healthcare-Data-Breach-Trends.pdf

[2] Ratchinsky, K. (2015, November 5). *IDC releases top 10 predictions for healthcare and IT is in the driver's seat*. Retrieved from http://www.healthcareitnews.com/blog/idc-releases-top-10-predictions-healthcare-it-drivers-seat

[3] Smith, M. (2014, October 3). *Medical ID theft: How scammers use records to steal your identity*. Retrieved from http://www.makeuseof.com/tag/medical-id-theft-scammers-use-records-steal-identity/

[4] Smith, M. (2014, October 3). *Medical ID theft: How scammers use records to steal your identity*. Retrieved from http://www.makeuseof.com/tag/medical-id-theft-scammers-use-records-steal-identity/

[5] Kuchler, H. (2015, June 17). *Patient records are target for cyber crooks*. Retrieved from http://www.ft.com/cms/s/0/20046010-e1cb-11e4-bb7f-00144feab7de.html#axzz3u1yOYeWL

[6] Lowes, R. *Stolen EHR charts sell for $50 each on black market*. Retrieved from http://www.medscape.com/viewarticle/824192

[7] Lowes, R. *Stolen EHR charts sell for $50 each on black market*. Retrieved from http://www.medscape.com/viewarticle/824192

NOTABLE HEALTHCARE BREACHES

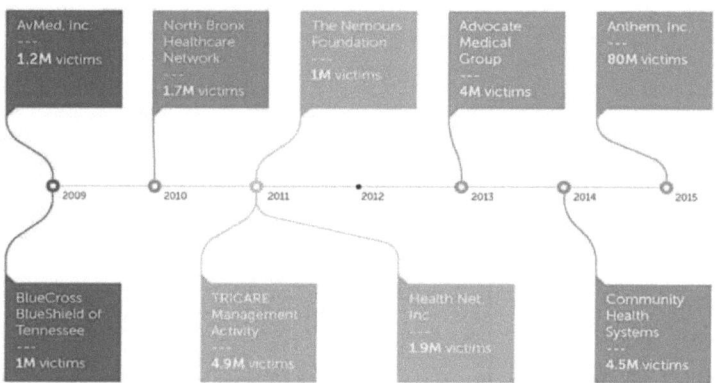

Figure 1: Notable data breaches in healthcare between 2009 and 2015
Source: InfoSec institute- http://resources.infosecinstitute.com/hackers-selling-healthcare-data-in-the-black-market/

Three underlying reasons for cyber attackers to hack health data include: lack of infrastructural security within the healthcare organization, shelf life of medical data, and the Social Security Number, which is particularly valuable in an identity theft.[8] It is intriguing that medical identity theft can impact not just victim's financial stability but can potentially put a patient's life under risk as victims of medical identity theft may receive the wrong type of care due to tampered medical files.[9] That said, it is important for healthcare organizations to implement best security practices to keep the sanctity of patients' records secure and intact.

While it's relatively easy to spot a credit card breach, the process of divining the provenance of stolen healthcare record, however, is not as straight forward.[10] The credit card industry has been combatting this threat long enough to have a streamlined process in place for dealing with

---

[8] Kossman, S. (2015, April 15). *Healthcare data breaches: Why you should be concerned.* Retrieved from http://blogs.creditcards.com/2015/04/health-care-data-breaches-why-you-should-be-concerned.php

[9] Weisman, S. (2015, July 25). *Another healthcare data breach.* Retrieved from http://www.usatoday.com/story/money/personalfinance/2015/07/24/steve-weisman-health-care-data-breach/30593661/

[10] Garrubba, T. (2014, November 10). *5 ways health data breaches are far worse than financial ones.* Retrieved from http://www.govhealthit.com/news/5-ways-health-data-breaches-are-far-worse-financial-ones

stolen information, but this is a new territory for healthcare.[11] An experiment conducted by Bitglass in April 2015 transmitted a few synthesized fake names, Social Security Numbers, and health record information through the company's proxy, which automatically watermarked the file.[12] Complexity to track a medical data breach is well simulated in **Figure 2.**

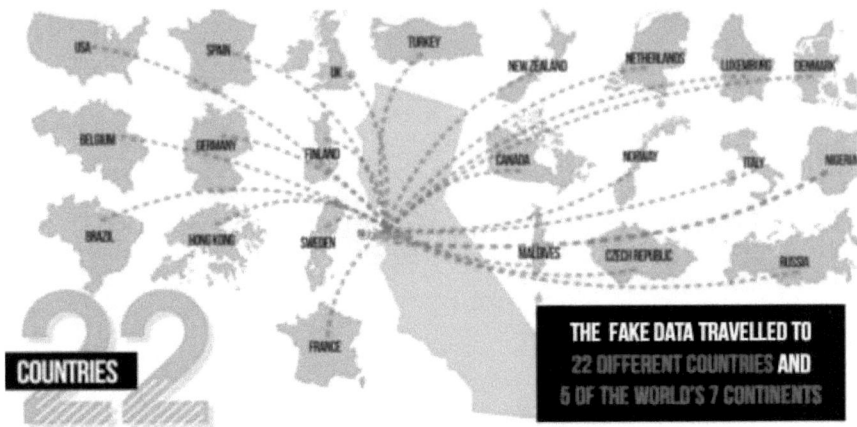

Figure 2: Complexity of a medical data breach
Source: Bitglass- http://krebsonsecurity.com/2015/04/a-day-in-the-life-of-a-stolen-healthcare-

Cybersecurity in healthcare is indeed alarming. It's little wonder why cybersecurity is the leading concern among health-IT decision makers. To get these security holes patched, healthcare facilities must identify potential risks, take appropriate actions, and improve diligence on revamping systems to prevent data theft.

This paper focuses on the need for better security controls taking into account numerous breaches and threat landscapes the healthcare sector in the United States is currently facing. At the outset, this paper provides insights into preparedness of healthcare organizations against potential breach threats, state-wise percentage analysis of healthcare data breach, and cloud technology as a solution for protection of data.

---

[11] Garrubba, T. (2014, November 10). *5 ways health data breaches are far worse than financial ones*. Retrieved from http://www.govhealthit.com/news/5-ways-health-data-breaches-are-far-worse-financial-ones

[12] Krebs, B. (2015, April 15). *A day in the life of a stolen healthcare record*. Retrieved from http://krebsonsecurity.com/2015/04/a-day-in-the-life-of-a-stolen-healthcare-record/

Hariesh Rajasekar

Arguments:

Data breaches in healthcare: Can customers' data be better protected by their healthcare institution?

Healthcare data remains to be a cyber crook's ideal target given its lucrative economic value, vulnerability of healthcare's cybersecurity system, and the ease of stealing medical information due to lack of infrastructural security within the industry.[13] Although the digital and technological revolution is shaping the future of connected care, the transition of U.S. healthcare to move their medical records to digital space has made the protected health information more available to skilled hackers.[14] The increasing cyber threats have been attributed to the ease of stealing medical information making it worth the trouble for hackers.[15] With hackers honing in on healthcare data, cyber threats on healthcare organizations have sharply increased by 100% between 2009 and 2013, and 72% between 2013 and 2014.[16] The aggressive and targeted cyber-attacks affecting the healthcare industry has now made cybersecurity a top business priority for healthcare organizations.

The puzzle to implement successful security practices from banking into healthcare has not been addressed, despite the track record of software and tools like total fraud protection, Kerberos, two factor authentication, detect-ID, and pretty good privacy (PGP).[17,18,19] Banks have stepped up their online security by incorporating advanced encryption technologies for secure transactions while health insurers and hospitals have not taken security seriously.[20] Funds are typically allocated by healthcare organizations for new machines and noteworthy physicians who drive more patients and have a direct impact on profits, while neglecting

---

[13] Kuchler, H. (2015, June 17). *Patient records are target for cyber crooks.* Retrieved from http://www.ft.com/cms/s/0/20046010-e1cb-11e4-bb7f-00144feab7de.html#axzz3u1yOYeWL

[14] Ponemon Institute. (2011, March). *Second annual survey on medical identity theft.* Retrieved from http://www.experian.com/assets/data-breach/white-papers/second-annual-survey-medical-idenity-theft.pdf

[15] Kossman, S. (2015, April 15). *Healthcare data breaches: Why you should be concerned.* Retrieved from http://blogs.creditcards.com/2015/04/health-care-data-breaches-why-you-should-be-concerned.php

[16] Ashiq, J.A. (2015, July 27). *Hackers selling healthcare data in the black market.* Retrieved from http://resources.infosecinstitute.com/hackers-selling-healthcare-data-in-the-black-market/

[17] Mathew, J. (2014, November). Hackers target medical records as electronic data becomes less lucrative. *International Business Times.* Retrieved from http://www.ibtimes.co.uk/hackers-target-medical-records-electronic-data-becomes-less-lucrative-1476043

[18] Yang, Y. J. (1997). The security of electronic banking. *National information.*

[19]Claessens, J., Dem, V., De Cock, D., Preneel, B., & Vandewalle, J. (2002). On the security of today's online electronic banking systems. *Computers & Security,* 21(3), 253-265.

[20] Ashiq, J.A. (2015, July 27). *Hackers selling healthcare data in the black market.* Retrieved from http://resources.infosecinstitute.com/hackers-selling-healthcare-data-in-the-black-market/

security.[21] Healthcare organization's IT budget percentage dedicated to information security is shown in the **Figure 3.**

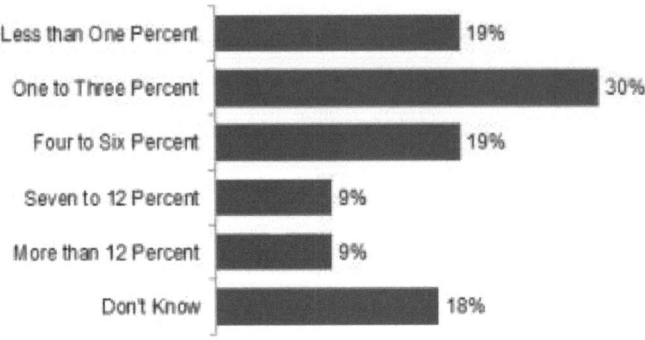

Figure 3: Percentage of IT budget dedicated to information security by healthcare organizations
Source: http://s3.amazonaws.com/rdcms-
himss/files/production/public/2013_HIMSS_Security_Survey.pdf

Many healthcare organizations neither perform encryption of records within the internal networks nor use encryption of data at rest and transit.[22] HIPAA addresses a number of patient privacy issues but doesn't require encryption of people's data.[22]

Security tools used by hospitals to defend data theft have changed since 2008 and is a positive change (**Figure 4**). Use of encryption, in transit and at rest, is also in the uptick. Survey respondents seem to agree that the traditional defensive weapon in use will likely not be helpful to defend them from the cyber-attacks of tomorrow.[23] More sophisticated and heuristics tools are thus required to aid in successful cyber defense in the future.

---

[21] Mundis, A. (2015, October). *Why healthcare data is becoming so valuable*. Retrieved from
http://www.resource1electronics.com/assets/increasing-value-of-health-information.pdf

[22] Ashiq, J.A. (2015, July 27). *Hackers selling healthcare data in the black market*. Retrieved from
http://resources.infosecinstitute.com/hackers-selling-healthcare-data-in-the-black-market/

[23] Miliard, M. (2015, November 12). *Cybersecurity strategies evolving in face of big risk*. Retrieved from
http://www.healthcareitnews.com/news/cybersecurity-strategies-evolving-face-big-risk

Top Security Tools	Count	Percent
Top Security Tools 2008 (N=155)		
Firewalls	153	98.7%
User access controls	147	94.8%
Audit logs	133	85.8%
Disaster recovery	130	83.9%
Wireless security protocols	126	81.3%
Top Security Tools 2015 (N=297)		
Antivirus/malware	258	86.9%
Firewalls	253	85.2%
Data encryption (data at rest)	208	70.0%
Data encryption (data in transit)	205	69.0%
Audit logs of each access to patient health and financial records	190	64.0%

Figure 4: A comparison of tools used by hospitals to defend data breaches in 2008 and 2015[23]
Source: http://www.healthcareitnews.com/news/cybersecurity-strategies-evolving-face-big-risk

Cyber security experts recommend that encryption of data would not be a 100% solution and will also require features like application and network security, multi-factor authentication, and data breach response plans that have often been overlooked for long.[24] Getting electronic medical devices patched and encrypting portable devices are other recommendations. A layered or **'defense in depth approach'** is the need of the hour as it would give the defenders sufficient time to identify the breach, delay the attackers and ultimately prevent the attack in order to keep the most upscale assets safe.[25] **Figure 5** shows some of the common errors that health organizations commit in conducting a risk assessment. Data protection strategy against medical data breach still remains **'a solution in search of a problem'** and no magic bullet has yet been proposed.

---

[24] Ashiq, J.A. (2015, July 27). *Hackers selling healthcare data in the black market.* Retrieved from http://resources.infosecinstitute.com/hackers-selling-healthcare-data-in-the-black-market/

[25] Bowen, C. (2015, July 8). *The seedy underworld of medical data trafficking.* Retrieved from http://www.healthcareitnews.com/blog/seedy-underworld-medical-data-trafficking

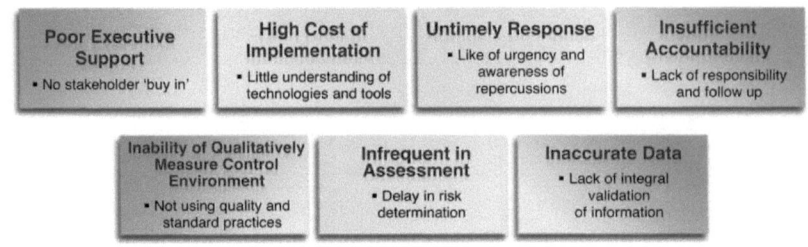

Figure 5: Errors committed by healthcare organizations in conducting a risk assessment
Source: https://lunarline.com/Healthcare-Security

Breaches by type: How the data is lost?

U.S. Department of Health & Human Services- Office for Civil Rights maintains a breach portal that requires healthcare organizations to report breaches of unsecured protected health information affecting 500 or more individuals, according to HITECH Act, section 13402(e)(4).[26] Seven types of breaches as classified by U.S. Department of Health & Human Services- Office for Civil Rights includes, hacking/IT incident, improper disposal, loss, others, theft, unauthorized access/disclosure, and unknown.[27] Although hacking is a form of theft, theft of data in this context accounts to those robbed or stolen personal devices.[28]

When there is an air of mystery about the threat landscape of cyber-attacks in health data breach, recent studies expatiating the pervasiveness of data breaches that result from loss or stolen computers, desktops, hard drives, back up tapes, PDA's, and other portable devices containing unencrypted personal information have eclipsed data lost due to cyber-attacks.[29,30]

A report by Bitglass in 2014 suggests that, 68% of the data breaches accounted to loss or theft and only a meagre 23% due to hacking.[31]

---

[26] https://ocrportal.hhs.gov/ocr/breach/breach_report.jsf

[27] https://ocrportal.hhs.gov/ocr/breach/breach_report.jsf

[28] https://ocrportal.hhs.gov/ocr/breach/breach_report.jsf

[29] Pennic, J. (2014, November). 68% of healthcare data breaches due to device loss or theft, not hacking. *Insightful coverage of healthcare technology*. Retrieved from http://hitconsultant.net/2014/11/04/healthcare-data-breaches-device-theft-loss/

[30] Hourihan, C., & Cline, B. (2012, December). A look back: U.S. healthcare data breach trends. *HITRUST*. Retrieved from https://hitrustalliance.net/content/uploads/2014/05/HITRUST-Report-U.S.-Healthcare-Data-Breach-Trends.pdf

[31] Bitglass. (2014). *The 2014 bitglass healthcare breach report*. Retrieved from http://pages.bitglass.com/rs/bitglass/images/WP-Healthcare-Report-2014.pdf

Raw data about breach report results (**2009-2015**) available in the U.S. Department of Health & Human Services- Office for Civil Rights breach portal was utilized for an infographic analysis (**using Microsoft Excel, SPSS, and Meta- Chart** (https://www.meta-chart.com/)) to explore,

- Percentage of data breaches by type
- State-wise percentage analysis of data breaches in healthcare and
- Location of breached information

Results of the analysis are shown in the **Figure 6, 7 and 8**.

Table 1 displays top 5 states that accounts for most number of medical data breaches.

Table 2, on the other hand, displays top 5 states that accounts for least number of medical data breaches.

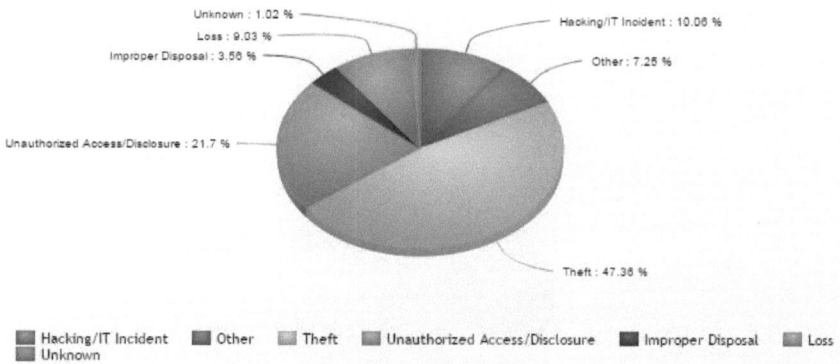

Figure 6: Percentage of data breaches by type
Data source: https://ocrportal.hhs.gov/ocr/breach/breach_report.jsf

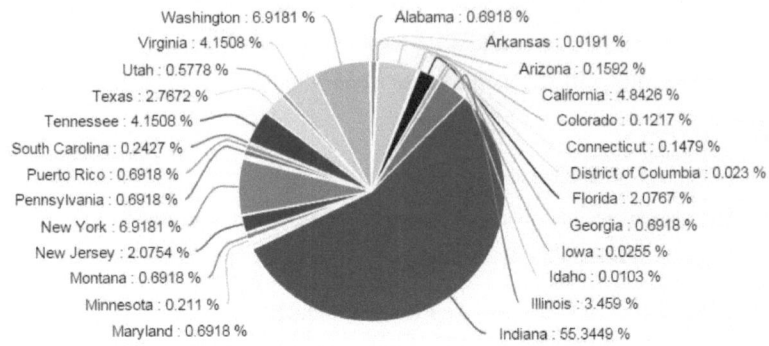

Figure 7: State-wise percentage analysis of data breaches in healthcare
Data source: https://ocrportal.hhs.gov/ocr/breach/breach_report.jsf

An interactive **Figure 7** is available at,

https://www.meta-chart.com/share/state-wise-percentage-analysis-of-data-breaches-in-healthcare

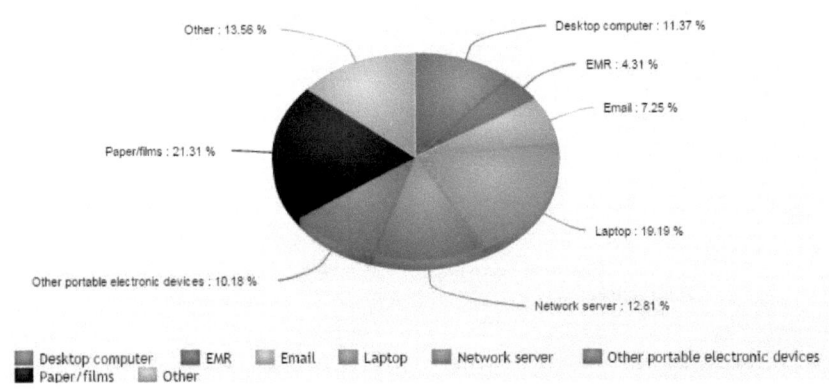

Figure 8: Location of breached information
Data source: https://ocrportal.hhs.gov/ocr/breach/breach_report.jsf

Table 1: Top 5 states that accounts for most number of medical data breaches
Data source: https://ocrportal.hhs.gov/ocr/breach/breach_report.jsf

Rank	State	Percentage (%)
1	Indiana (IN)	55.3449
2	Washington (WA) and New York (NY)	6.9181
3	California (CA)	4.8426
4	Virginia (VA) and Tennessee (TN)	4.1508
5	Illinois (IL)	3.4590

Table 2: Top 5 states that accounts for least number of medical data breaches
Data source: https://ocrportal.hhs.gov/ocr/breach/breach_report.jsf

Rank	State	Percentage (%)
1	Hawaii (HI)	0.0004
2	Alaska (AK)	0.0005
3	Delaware (DE)	0.0013
4	Vermont (VT)	0.0017
5	North Carolina (NC)	0.0020

It is evident from the analysis that, the bitter truth is healthcare data is more likely to be robbed than hacked! This infographic analysis can in turn be correlated to patient's trust, which will potentially provide a lot of room for further studies and scholarly debates.

Cloud storage of medical data: Safe or sloppy?

E-cloud refers to storage of data to a remote device, often described as a storage system that's maintained by a third party.[32] With healthcare rapidly proceeding towards a digital-first environment, cloud computing is at the center of this transformation.

In a survey conducted by HIMSS Analytics on adoption of cloud computing in healthcare, it was found that 83% of healthcare organizations reported using some form of cloud-based

---

[32] Leymann, F. (2011). Cloud computing. *it-Information Technology Methoden und innovative Anwendungen der Informatik und Informationstechnik, 53*(4), 163-164.

services.[33] The major perceived benefit for adoption of cloud in healthcare is believed to offload a burdensome task from hospital IT departments allowing them to shift their focus and achieve goals on other components such as meaningful use, enhanced clinical support systems etc.[34] Current areas of cloud application in healthcare is shown in the **Figure 9.**

	Current Use	Planned Use	No Use	Total
Hosting of Clinical Applications and Data	43.6%	14.1%	42.3%	100.0%
Health Information Exchange	38.7%	20.0%	41.3%	100.0%
Backups and Disaster Recovery	35.1%	31.1%	33.7%	100.0%
Hosting of HR Applications and Data	34.9%	16.8%	48.3%	100.0%
Hosting Financial Applications and Data	32.9%	18.8%	48.3%	100.0%
Hosting Operational Applications and Data	27.7%	28.4%	43.9%	100.0%
Hosting of Archived Data	26.8%	38.9%	34.3%	100.0%
Hosting Back Office Applications and Data	22.1%	22.1%	55.8%	100.0%
Managed Services	22.1%	17.4%	60.5%	100.0%
Hosting Communications Services	20.3%	20.3%	59.4%	100.0%
Server Virtualization	14.9%	12.2%	72.9%	100.0%
Desktop Virtualization	8.1%	14.2%	77.7%	100.0%
Virtual Networks	6.1%	8.8%	85.1%	100.0%
Accountable Care Organization	6.0%	13.5%	80.5%	100.0%
Identity Management	2.0%	8.1%	89.9%	100.0%
Timely Provisioning or Deprovisioning Accounts	2.0%	6.1%	91.9%	100.0%

N = 150

Figure 9: Current areas of cloud application in healthcare
Source: Forbes- http://www.forbes.com/sites/louiscolumbus/2014/07/17/83-of-healthcare-organizations-are-using-cloud-based-apps-today/

Majority of hospitals and healthcare systems still use client-server systems which is predominantly vulnerable to data breaches caused by technology deficiencies, theft, and insider misconduct.[35] Cloud Standards Customer Council exclaims that cloud-computing can be

---

[33] Columbus, L. (2014, July 17). *83% of healthcare organizations are using cloud-based apps today*. Retrieved from http://www.forbes.com/sites/louiscolumbus/2014/07/17/83-of-healthcare-organizations-are-using-cloud-based-apps-today/

[34] Cloud Standards Customer Council. (2012, November). *Impact of cloud computing on healthcare*. Retrieved from http://www.cloud-council.org/cscchealthcare110512.pdf

[35] Cloud Standards Customer Council. (2012, November). *Impact of cloud computing on healthcare*. Retrieved from http://www.cloud-council.org/cscchealthcare110512.pdf

custom designed to make the defense safer than traditional client-server systems against the prevailing causes of healthcare data breaches.[36]

A web-based secure private cloud is a solution to insider threat that accounts for 68% of medical data breaches.[37] This should eventually protect the data from disgruntled employees and patient-record snoopers. The difference between secure private cloud and client-server systems is the proximity of sensitive data to those who might misuse it or in other terms the number of people who have access to the portals.[38]

Numerous benefits are listed for adoption of cloud computing in healthcare and cloud technologies can significantly facilitate these trends.[39] However, issues related to service reliability, integration and interoperability, and data portability, continue to be challenges to leverage cloud computing for healthcare.[40] Challenges relating to legislation in the U.S. and HIPAA are other barriers to adoption of cloud technology.[41] One important issue pertaining to U.S. legislation and HIPAA towards cloud storage of medical data is that data is not supposed to leave this country (U.S), although it is known that storing data abroad would save huge overhead cost spent for labor, electricity etc.[42]

The prediction by International Data Corporation for healthcare cloud creation to become a top market strategy for tech providers and industrial companies in 2018 makes cloud storage and data security, almost en masse.[43]

---

[36] Cloud Standards Customer Council. (2012, November). *Impact of cloud computing on healthcare*. Retrieved from http://www.cloud-council.org/cscchealthcare110512.pdf

[37] Cloud Standards Customer Council. (2012, November). *Impact of cloud computing on healthcare*. Retrieved from http://www.cloud-council.org/cscchealthcare110512.pdf

[38] Cloud Standards Customer Council. (2012, November). *Impact of cloud computing on healthcare*. Retrieved from http://www.cloud-council.org/cscchealthcare110512.pdf

[39] Columbus, L. (2014, July 17). *83% of healthcare organizations are using cloud-based apps today*. Retrieved from http://www.forbes.com/sites/louiscolumbus/2014/07/17/83-of-healthcare-organizations-are-using-cloud-based-apps-today/

[40] Cloud Standards Customer Council. (2012, November). *Impact of cloud computing on healthcare*. Retrieved from http://www.cloud-council.org/cscchealthcare110512.pdf

[41] Annas, G. J. (2003). HIPAA regulations-a new era of medical-record privacy? *New England Journal of Medicine*, 348(15), 1486-1490.

[42] Cloud Standards Customer Council. (2012, November). *Impact of cloud computing on healthcare*. Retrieved from http://www.cloud-council.org/cscchealthcare110512.pdf

[43] Ratchinsky, K. (2015, November 5). *IDC releases top 10 predictions for healthcare and IT is in the driver's seat*. Retrieved from http://www.healthcareitnews.com/blog/idc-releases-top-10-predictions-healthcare-it-drivers-seat

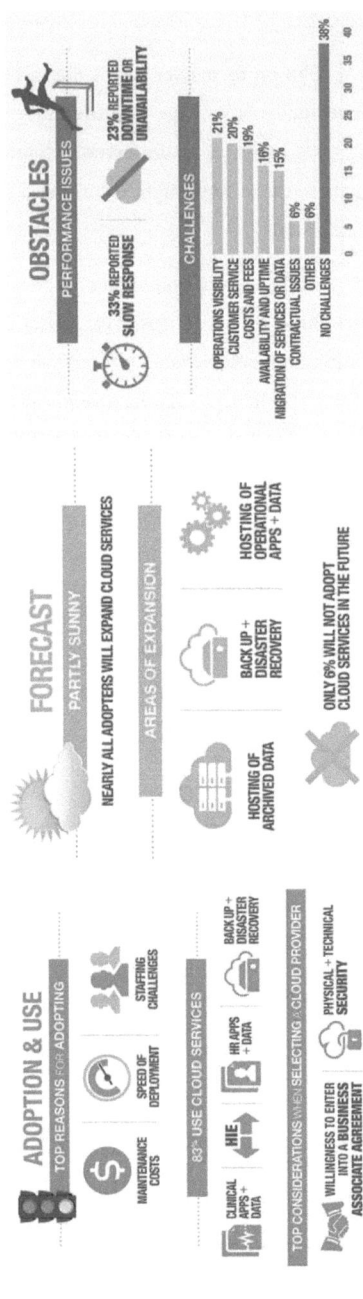

Figure 10: Cloud technology in healthcare- An insight

Figure 10 provides an insight into the possibilities cloud technology can enable in healthcare, its barrier to adoption and forecast.

Source: http://www.forbes.com/sites/louiscolumbus/2014/07/17/83-of-healthcare-organizations-are-using-cloud-based-apps-today/

The best defense I believe for a healthcare organization is to find a cloud partner that has been successful and determined in preventing the cyber thieves of today. Cloud is a process, not a technology revolution. From what it looks now, it's going to get cloudier!

Conclusion:

Economics of healthcare data theft, which was previously overlooked, has now become the prime attention of hackers and is widely regarded as **'The triple crown of stolen data'**.[44] The lack of infrastructural security within the healthcare industry have made things simpler for hackers to gain access to and involve in impersonate purposes.[45]

The two most recent breaches at Anthem, and Excellus Blue Cross Blue Shield has exposed the enormous gap in data security.[46,47] With a whopping 44% of data breaches that healthcare and other related organizations contribute to, it is important to diligently examine factors that make medical data theft a growing problem.[48] HIPAA, for sure, may have a positive impact, but it certainly isn't keeping the healthcare organizations and hospitals from becoming a poster child for stolen personal information.

Unlike a credit card theft where banks will most likely cancel the charges, an extrapolated out-of-pocket expenses per victim of medical ID theft is $18,660.[49] Such report on healthcare data breach make credit card theft look like child's play.

Security tools used by hospitals to defend data theft have changed since 2008, with encryption technology in the uptick.[50] Although adoption of cloud computing in healthcare has grown tremendously, web-based secure private cloud, and cloud-based client server system, that show

[44] Mathew, J. (2014, November 22). *Hackers target medical records as electronic data becomes lucrative.* Retrieved from http://www.ibtimes.co.uk/hackers-target-medical-records-electronic-data-becomes-less-lucrative-1476043

[45] Kuchler, H. (2015, June 17). *Patient records are target for cyber crooks.* Retrieved from http://www.ft.com/cms/s/0/20046010-e1cb-11e4-bb7f-00144feab7de.html#axzz3u1yOYeWL

[46] Yasin, R. (2015, September 10). *Another healthcare insurer, Excellus BCBS, hit with mega-breach.* Retrieved from http://www.darkreading.com/attacks-breaches/another-healthcare-insurer-excellus-bcbs-hit-with-mega-breach/d/d-id/1322142

[47] Hiltzik, M. (2015, March 6). Anthem is warning consumers about its huge data breach. Here's a translation. Retrieved from http://www.latimes.com/business/hiltzik/la-fi-mh-anthem-is-warning-consumers-20150306-column.html

[48] Bitglass. (2014). *The 2014 bitglass healthcare breach report.* Retrieved from http://pages.bitglass.com/rs/bitglass/images/WP-Healthcare-Report-2014.pdf

[49] Bitglass. (2014). *The 2014 bitglass healthcare breach report.* Retrieved from http://pages.bitglass.com/rs/bitglass/images/WP-Healthcare-Report-2014.pdf

[50] Miliard, M. (2015, November 12). *Cybersecurity strategies evolving in face of big risk.* Retrieved from http://www.healthcareitnews.com/news/cybersecurity-strategies-evolving-face-big-risk

promise in protection of medical data, have however, not started to trend yet.[51] It is observed from the analysis that, healthcare organizations are preparing for the level of sophistication associated with the attacks that will be coming at them.

Reports of breaches against healthcare organizations, large and small, continue to rise. Results of this paper show that health care's critical information assets are poorly protected and are often compromised. Cyber crooks are well connected, organized, and have better technology. That said, it's high time that diligence on revamping systems to prevent data theft becomes a top priority for healthcare sector!

---

[51] Cloud Standards Customer Council. (2012, November). *Impact of cloud computing on healthcare*. Retrieved from http://www.cloud-council.org/cscchealthcare110512.pdf

Hariesh Rajasekar

References:

Hourihan, C., Cline, B. (2012, December). *A look back: U.S. healthcare data breach trends*. Retrieved from https://hitrustalliance.net/content/uploads/2014/05/HITRUST-Report-U.S.-Healthcare-Data-Breach-Trends.pdf

Ratchinsky, K. (2015, November 5). *IDC releases top 10 predictions for healthcare and IT is in the driver's seat*. Retrieved from http://www.healthcareitnews.com/blog/idc-releases-top-10-predictions-healthcare-it-drivers-seat

Smith, M. (2014, October 3). *Medical ID theft: How scammers use records to steal your identity*. Retrieved from http://www.makeuseof.com/tag/medical-id-theft-scammers-use-records-steal-identity/

Kuchler, H. (2015, June 17). *Patient records are target for cyber crooks*. Retrieved from http://www.ft.com/cms/s/0/20046010-e1cb-11e4-bb7f-00144feab7de.html#axzz3u1yOYeWL

Lowes, R. *Stolen EHR charts sell for $50 each on black market*. Retrieved from http://www.medscape.com/viewarticle/824192

Kossman, S. (2015, April 15). *Healthcare data breaches: Why you should be concerned*. Retrieved from http://blogs.creditcards.com/2015/04/health-care-data-breaches-why-you-should-be-concerned.php

Weisman, S. (2015, July 25). *Another healthcare data breach*. Retrieved from http://www.usatoday.com/story/money/personalfinance/2015/07/24/steve-weisman-health-care-data-breach/30593661/

Garrubba, T. (2014, November 10). *5 ways health data breaches are far worse than financial ones*. Retrieved from http://www.govhealthit.com/news/5-ways-health-data-breaches-are-far-worse-financial-ones

Krebs, B. (2015, April 15). A day in the life of a stolen healthcare record. Retrieved from http://krebsonsecurity.com/2015/04/a-day-in-the-life-of-a-stolen-healthcare-record/

Ponemon Institute. (2011, March). *Second annual survey on medical identity theft*. Retrieved from http://www.experian.com/assets/data-breach/white-papers/second-annual-survey-medical-idenity-theft.pdf

Ashiq, J.A. (2015, July 27). *Hackers selling healthcare data in the black market*. Retrieved from http://resources.infosecinstitute.com/hackers-selling-healthcare-data-in-the-black-market/

Mathew, J. (2014, November). Hackers target medical records as electronic data becomes less lucrative. *International Business Times*. Retrieved from http://www.ibtimes.co.uk/hackers-target-medical-records-electronic-data-becomes-less-lucrative-1476043

Yang, Y. J. (1997). The security of electronic banking. *National information*.

Claessens, J., Dem, V., De Cock, D., Preneel, B., & Vandewalle, J. (2002). On the security of today's online electronic banking systems. *Computers & Security*, 21(3), 253-265.

Mundis, A. (2015, October). *Why healthcare data is becoming so valuable*. Retrieved from http://www.resource1electronics.com/assets/increasing-value-of-health-information.pdf

Miliard, M. (2015, November 12). *Cybersecurity strategies evolving in face of big risk*. Retrieved from http://www.healthcareitnews.com/news/cybersecurity-strategies-evolving-face-big-risk

Bowen, C. (2015, July 8). *The seedy underworld of medical data trafficking*. Retrieved from http://www.healthcareitnews.com/blog/seedy-underworld-medical-data-trafficking

https://ocrportal.hhs.gov/ocr/breach/breach_report.jsf

Pennic, J. (2014, November). 68% of healthcare data breaches due to device loss or theft, not hacking. *Insightful coverage of healthcare technology*. Retrieved from http://hitconsultant.net/2014/11/04/healthcare-data-breaches-device-theft-loss/

Hourihan, C., & Cline, B. (2012, December). A look back: U.S. healthcare data breach trends. *HITRUST*. Retrieved from https://hitrustalliance.net/content/uploads/2014/05/HITRUST-Report-U.S.-Healthcare-Data-Breach-Trends.pdf

Bitglass. (2014). *The 2014 bitglass healthcare breach report*. Retrieved from http://pages.bitglass.com/rs/bitglass/images/WP-Healthcare-Report-2014.pdf

Leymann, F. (2011). Cloud computing. *it-Information Technology Methoden und innovative Anwendungen der Informatik und Informationstechnik, 53*(4), 163-164.

Columbus, L. (2014, July 17). *83% of healthcare organizations are using cloud-based apps today*. Retrieved from http://www.forbes.com/sites/louiscolumbus/2014/07/17/83-of-healthcare-organizations-are-using-cloud-based-apps-today/

Cloud Standards Customer Council. (2012, November). *Impact of cloud computing on healthcare*. Retrieved from http://www.cloud-council.org/cscchealthcare110512.pdf

Annas, G. J. (2003). HIPAA regulations-a new era of medical-record privacy? *New England Journal of Medicine, 348*(15), 1486-1490.

Mathew, J. (2014, November 22). *Hackers target medical records as electronic data becomes lucrative*. Retrieved from http://www.ibtimes.co.uk/hackers-target-medical-records-electronic-data-becomes-less-lucrative-1476043

Yasin, R. (2015, September 10). *Another healthcare insurer, Excellus BCBS, hit with mega-breach*. Retrieved from http://www.darkreading.com/attacks-breaches/another-healthcare-insurer-excellus-bcbs-hit-with-mega-breach/d/d-id/1322142

Hiltzik, M. (2015, March 6). Anthem is warning consumers about its huge data breach. Here's a translation. Retrieved from http://www.latimes.com/business/hiltzik/la-fi-mh-anthem-is-warning-consumers-20150306-column.html

YOUR KNOWLEDGE HAS VALUE

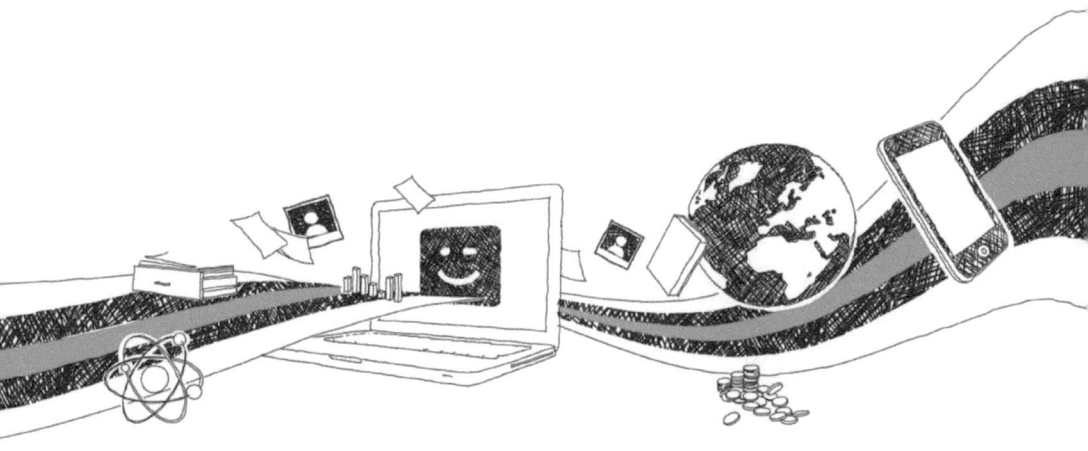

- We will publish your bachelor's and
  master's thesis, essays and papers

- Your own eBook and book -
  sold worldwide in all relevant shops

- Earn money with each sale

Upload your text at www.GRIN.com
and publish for free

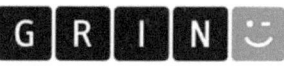